Alicia Margarita Lopez Diaz de Cabrera

Working Conditions and Job Satisfaction

Alicia Margarita Lopez Diaz de Cabrera

Working Conditions and Job Satisfaction

of the Surgical Center Health Care Personnel

ScienciaScripts

Imprint
Any brand names and product names mentioned in this book are subject to trademark, brand or patent protection and are trademarks or registered trademarks of their respective holders. The use of brand names, product names, common names, trade names, product descriptions etc. even without a particular marking in this work is in no way to be construed to mean that such names may be regarded as unrestricted in respect of trademark and brand protection legislation and could thus be used by anyone.

Cover image: www.ingimage.com

This book is a translation from the original published under ISBN 978-613-9-44228-7.

Publisher:
Sciencia Scripts
is a trademark of
Dodo Books Indian Ocean Ltd. and OmniScriptum S.R.L publishing group

120 High Road, East Finchley, London, N2 9ED, United Kingdom
Str. Armeneasca 28/1, office 1, Chisinau MD-2012, Republic of Moldova, Europe
Printed at: see last page
ISBN: 978-620-6-87311-2

Table of Contents :

NATIONAL UNIVERSITY OF TRUJILLO

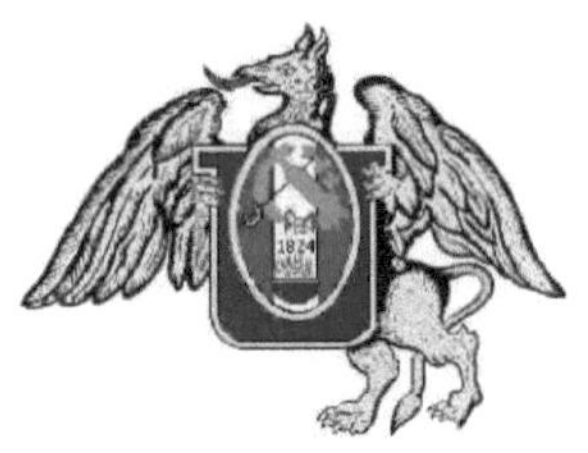

WORKING CONDITIONS AND JOB SATISFACTION OF THE HEALTH PERSONNEL OF THE SURGICAL CENTER - TRUJILLO REGIONAL TEACHING HOSPITAL". REGIONAL TEACHING HOSPITAL OF TRUJILLO".

ALICIA MARGARITA LÓPEZ DÍAZ DE CABRERA.

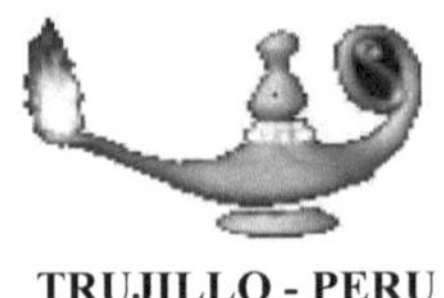

TRUJILLO - PERU

DEDICATION

To the forger of my path, God the Heavenly Father, who always accompanies me and guides my steps to improve my life.

To my mother, María Perpetua, because you always instilled in me the desire to excel, the effort, the responsibility to achieve life's goals; I will be eternally grateful for your immense love, even though you are no longer present.

To my husband Eduar, for his support and understanding so that I can continue to improve myself. To my children: Enver, Maryan and Danny for their motivation to continue studying regardless of life's adversities.

THANK YOU

To Almighty God for allowing me to overcome all obstacles in order to reach the goal of becoming a nurse specialist.

To my teachers of the Second Nursing Specialty of the National University of Trujillo, Surgical Center Mention; who from the beginning have been kind enough to offer us their knowledge with patience and dedication.

Yaneth Reyes Guzmán who was my advisor, to whom I express my gratitude for supporting me with her suggestions in the elaboration, correction and completion of the present work.

To my friends from the Second Specialty: Laura, Rocío, Marilia, Nelly, Cinthia; with whom I have shared, learned and overcome different situations in order to become specialists.

Finally, I would like to thank the staff of the Hospital Regional Docente de Trujillo, where I work, for supporting me in developing this project and finishing my thesis report.

SUMMARY

The present research study is quantitative, descriptive-correlational and cross-sectional. It was conducted with the health personnel of the surgical center during the months of January and February 2016, whose objective was to determine the relationship between working conditions and the level of job satisfaction. The sample population consisted of 51 people including physicians, nurses and nursing technicians who met the established inclusion criteria. The information was obtained through the instruments: Evaluation of working conditions and for job satisfaction the Font Roja Questionnaire which are valid and validated. The results obtained were tabulated and presented in simple and double-entry statistical tables. The information obtained was processed using the IBM statistical program, SPSS STATISTIC 23. From the results it is concluded that there are acceptable working conditions, which have a significant relationship with the average level of job satisfaction.

***Key words**: Working conditions, Job satisfaction.*

ABSTRACT

The present research study is of a quantitative, descriptive-correlational and cross-sectional type. It was carried out with the health personnel of the surgical center during the months of January and February 2016, whose objective was to determine the relationship that exists between working conditions and the level of job satisfaction. The sample population consisted of 51 people among doctors, nurses and nursing technicians who met the established inclusion criteria. The information was obtained through the instruments: Assessment of working conditions and for job satisfaction the Font Roja Questionnaire which are valid and validated. The results obtained were tabulated and presented in simple and double entry statistical tables. The information obtained was processed using the statistical program IBM, SPSS STATISTIC 23. From the results it is concluded that there are acceptable work conditions, the same ones that have a significant relationship with the average level of job satisfaction.

Keywords: Working conditions, Job satisfaction.

Chapter 1

I. INTRODUCTION

According to the International Labor Organization (ILO), 2009, the importance of investment in human capital to increase productivity and international competitiveness is now recognized and democracy has deepened through greater integration and social cohesion, to which social and labor protection contribute (Economic Commission for Latin America and the Caribbean, 2009).

Finally, tripartite initiatives have emerged from the dialogue between social actors (employers and workers) that aim to address the crisis by preventing the costs of adjustment from falling disproportionately on workers in terms of unemployment, lower wages and loss of other labor rights (Anaya, 2010).

Job satisfaction has become one of the main objectives of study for organizations. The contribution of disciplines such as psychology, sociology, administration and very recently nursing, have allowed the development of research studies that indicate that the satisfaction of people with their work is one of the basic determinants for the productivity of these organizations (Contreras, 2013).

Numerous studies show that the vast majority of personnel working in hospitals are not satisfied in their work environment; they feel that they have little control over their environment and feel that they are not valued for the work they do (Anaya, 2010).

An inadequate work environment can become a source of stress, negatively impacting an individual's job satisfaction and performance, since a person under conditions of dissatisfaction and family problems decreases his or her performance capacity (Anaya,

2010).

There are factors statistically associated with satisfaction that include the following: work shift: it seems that the morning shift is the one they feel most satisfied, they believe they have more possibilities of promotion, physical conditions of the workplace, possibilities of changing activities, relationships with colleagues of the same and different categories, compatibility of the schedule with personal life, opportunity for training and feeling integrated into the work team, feeling supported and valued by their superiors and valued by the rest of the colleagues, positively influences satisfaction (Anaya, 2010).

Job satisfaction is the attitude with which the worker faces his own job. This attitude, based on the beliefs and values that the worker develops about his own work, is determined jointly by the current characteristics of the job with the worker's perceptions of what it should be (Jaramillo & Mendoza, 2010).

Job satisfaction is a function of the discrepancies perceived by the individual between what he believes the job should give him and what he actually obtains as a product or gratification. It is the product of the comparison between the contributions made by the individual to the job and the product or result obtained. This same trend called equity also states that this satisfaction or dissatisfaction is a relative concept and depends on the comparisons made by the individual in terms of contributions and the results obtained by other individuals in their work environment or frame of reference (Jaramillo & Mendoza, 2010).

According to Spector (2002), job satisfaction is a subjective and individual perception resulting from an affective evaluation of people within an organization in relation to their work and the consequences derived from it. For several years, job satisfaction has been studied and discussed in different areas of knowledge such as psychology, sociology, administration and even nursing, where job satisfaction has been identified as a key indicator of performance, cost savings and quality of patient care (Cifuentes, 2012).

While job satisfaction responds to a positive emotional state resulting from the perception of work experiences and is, therefore, an important factor that conditions the individual's attitude towards his or her job, there are organizational and functional factors that can generate dissatisfaction in nursing personnel.

Frederick Herzberg (2010), argues that intrinsic and extrinsic factors are involved in the satisfaction or dissatisfaction of individuals in relation to their work. Among the former, he mentions the employee-job relationship, fulfillment, recognition, promotion, stimulating work and responsibility.

This same author argues that human beings feel truly satisfied with their work when they feel that it allows them to develop greater responsibility and experience mental and psychological growth. This allowed that in the late sixties and early seventies, improvements were made in the work that consisted of enriching it and improving the morale and performance of workers (Cardoso, 2013).

Back in the fifties of the last century, Abraham Maslow (1943), a humanist psychologist, established a hierarchy of needs whose satisfaction is vital, and nestled in the highest place are those that allow personal development. This hierarchy includes different aspects that influence satisfaction, such as physiological and security needs.

There are still organizations in which the employee is considered to be the *homo economicus* as already thought by the scientific school of the administration, and therefore, treat it as a burdensome cost and not as a resource to be developed and cared for, forgetting that people have interests, desires, expectations and needs, as contemplated by the theories of motivation, which were an important wake-up call in the job satisfaction research.

In health institutions, specifically in the hospital activity, there are factors or conditions that can affect the job satisfaction of their workers, which in turn can influence their level of individual and organizational performance (Hernandez, 2009).

THEORETICAL FRAMEWORK

Working conditions vary, according to different authors, and therefore the components of each of their categories of analysis; for this research, the concept taken up by Acosta was taken into account, according to which working conditions and the work environment are inherent to the work process and refer to "the set of factors that act on the individual in a work situation, determining his activity and causing a series of consequences both for the individual himself (human costs) and for the company (economic costs)" (García, Beltrán, & Daza, 2011).

Guerrero, who understands working conditions as "the total set of variables present during the performance of a task, was also taken into account.

It includes variables that characterize the task itself (work environment and work structuring), individual and personal variables, extra-work and psychosocial factors that may affect its development") (García, Beltrán, & Daza, 2011).

Finally, the definition formulated by the National University of Colombia was considered, which in its master's degree in Occupational Health and Safety contemplates working conditions as the set of intralaboral, extralaboral and individual factors that interact with the performance of the task determining the health-illness process of the workers and their working capacity (National University of Colombia, 2008).

This approach includes: individual conditions that are endogenous, inherent and intrinsic to the individual and make him or her unique and unrepeatable, since, in accordance with the diversity of the workforce, individual human characteristics make people different from one another.

However, some companies create stereotypes that attempt to group individuals into categories according to predominant characteristics;

In addition, the person throughout his or her life cycle is conditioned by hereditary, environmental, social and cultural factors; therefore, the analysis of his or her conditions was carried out taking into account various concepts contained in the theory.

In this sense, we can say: the working conditions that occur in daily work will greatly influence the health personnel to feel satisfied in performing their work, which is why we will mention job satisfaction in its various definitions.

Locke defines job satisfaction as: "a positive or pleasant emotional state resulting from the subjective perception of the work experiences of each subject". Spector defines it as a subjective and individual perception resulting from an affective evaluation that people make within an organization in relation to their work and the consequences derived from it (Contreras, 2013).

The concept of Job Satisfaction or job satisfaction has been widely studied from disciplines such as sociology and psychology. There have been many efforts aimed at the knowledge of the subject, based on the concern for the problems of work in societies, which have resulted in a considerable number of books and articles in fields other than social sciences.

During the 1930s, the first research studies on job satisfaction and the factors that could affect it were produced. By 1935 Hoppock published the first research where he made an in-depth analysis of satisfaction, finding that factors such as fatigue, monotony, working conditions and supervision, could influence job satisfaction (Cardoso, 2013).

In later studies, Herzberg suggested that man's real satisfaction with his job came from enriching the job, so that in this way he can develop greater responsibility and in turn experience mental and psychological growth (Contreras, 2013).

Later, towards the end of the 1960s and beginning of the 1970s, Locke (1976) defined job satisfaction as a "positive or pleasant emotional state of the subjective perception of the subject's work experiences" (Viamontes, 2010).

In other words, he considers Job Satisfaction as the product of the discrepancy between what the worker wants from his job and what he actually gets, mediated by the importance it has for the worker. In this sense, he proposes that the smaller the discrepancy between what the worker wants and what he gets, the greater the Job Satisfaction. By this date, 1970 and early 1980, nurses began to investigate mainly in the theoretical field of psychology and administration (Contreras, 2013).

Robbins, for his part, defines job satisfaction as the individual's general attitude towards his work, understanding that work is more than the obvious activities of handling documents, writing programming codes, waiting for customers or driving a vehicle. It also requires dealing with co-workers and bosses, obeying the rules and customs of the organization, meeting performance criteria, living in less than ideal working conditions, etc. (Robbins, 2004).

For Mottaz (1988), job satisfaction refers to an affective response that is the result of an evaluation of the work situation. While for Diez de Castro, García del Junco and Martín Jiménez, the concept of job satisfaction responds to an individual feeling that, in positive or negative terms, individuals experience in the course of their belonging to the organization when they compare the rewards they receive with those they consider they should receive and, even, with those they would like to obtain as compensation for the efforts they make in favor of the organization (Contreras, 2013).

For Loitegui, job satisfaction corresponds to a multidimensional construct that depends both on the individual characteristics of the subject and on the characteristics and specificities of the work performed. In this sense, job satisfaction depends on the interaction between two types of variables: the results achieved by the worker through the performance of his own work and how these results are perceived and experienced according to the characteristics and peculiarities of the worker's personality (Georgina, 2011).

For Alonso-Calderon, Ayora-Vivas, Bellás-Farré, and Eloy-García, (1999) job satisfaction is defined as the result of the appreciation that each individual makes of his job and that allows him to reach or admit the knowledge of its importance and responds to a positive or pleasant emotional state resulting from this subjective perception of work experiences and that are congruent or helpful in satisfying his needs (Calderon, 1999).

In general terms, when speaking of job satisfaction, elements related to perceptions, feelings or affective responses referred to work are included, which can be generalized or global and include all the factors described by the different authors, and on the other hand, it can be referred to one or some of the aspects or dimensions of work. Attempts have been made to explain job satisfaction from different theories; in most cases, motivational theories have been used to explain this phenomenon due to the central role that motivation plays in it.

There is less consensus among theorists as to which standards are relevant for the confrontation of work experiences. Some of the alternatives are the following: Comparison between needs and outcomes (Maslow's and McClelland's theory of needs).

Subjects continuously compare their current state of needs with the level of satisfaction they wish to obtain from their jobs. If the needs are not satisfied, a state of tension appears that makes workers dissatisfied; otherwise they will feel satisfied. Comparison with others (relative deprivation theory).

Individuals base their concept of justice on the confrontation of their own results with those obtained by other subjects in their work environment or frame of reference. Comparison of contributions/results (Adams' theory of fairness). The worker observes the efforts made by others in their work and the rewards they obtain and compares it with his situation. The only desirable condition is one in which such a comparison indicates equality. Comparison with the expected (Vroom's expectations theory).

Job satisfaction is a function of the discrepancies perceived by the individual between what he should give to his current job and what he actually obtains as a product or gratification. Comparison with values (Locke's value theory). Subjects make comparisons with their overall objectives or goals (what they want, desire, or value) in relation to the work experience.

The theories of motivation most commonly used by researchers to address the phenomenon of job satisfaction. Locke (1969), distinguishes three initial stages attributed to schools fundamentally oriented towards task design: The Physico-economic school, dating back to Taylor in 1911, and his idea of scientific organization of work, with an economic point of view coupled with a physiological point of view, which tries to address fatigue by seeking means to reduce it.

This trend remained central during the 1930s with studies on health and industrial fatigue showing the benefit of the role played by breaks, scheduling structure, etc.

Researchers introduce various stimulants into work processes, which are not directly useful for increasing production, but are indirectly useful because of their effect on job satisfaction.

The psychological or human relations school, which has its origin in the work of Elton (1933), his research on fatigue and absence of breaks in the textile industry, led him to note that factors such as links with management or group environments also played a role in employee attitudes and could be modified to some extent by psycho-social interventions.

This movement developed, in part, because of the proliferation, since the beginning of the Second World War, of leadership studies. Connections with both the hierarchical superior and the group were at the center of concerns.

The years 1955-1960 constitute the culminating period of the causal association between human relations and job satisfaction. The developmental school, born with the study of Herzberg *et al.* in 1959 and strongly linked to Maslow's theory of needs.

His Dual or Two-Factor theory is based on the idea that people have two kinds of needs: hygiene needs, which are related to the physical and psychological conditions in which they work, and motivational needs, which were conceived as being very similar to the higher needs Maslow spoke of in 1954 in his theory.

These two types of requirements are satisfied by different kinds of rewards. Hygiene needs are satisfied by the levels of certain conditions called hygienizing or dissatisfying factors, related to the context or environment in which the work is to be performed (extrinsic factors). On the other hand, motivational needs are satisfied by what they called motivating or satisfying factors, linked to the nature of the work itself (intrinsic factors).

Satisfying hygiene needs does not result in job satisfaction but only in the reduction or elimination of dissatisfaction. On the other hand, motivating factors, which satisfy the self-fulfillment needs of an individual at work, produce satisfaction when they are present, while when they are absent they produce the same "neutral state" associated with the presence of hygienizing factors.

These three schools of thought place the determinants of total satisfaction in different spheres. The physical-economic approach emphasizes adequate physical working conditions. The psychosocial approach focuses on the importance of effective supervision and cohesive work groups. The developmental perspective emphasizes the feelings of satisfied employees due to mentally demanding tasks. Job-related variables, (i.e., job characteristics, responsibilities assumed, amount of work, perceived control over procedures) are considered important in understanding job satisfaction, because these variables create an immediate and strong situational influence.

Abraham Maslow's theory (1943) states that the development of the human personality starts from a supreme need. As human beings who participate in all human needs, in this process of satisfaction and after having satisfied other physiological needs, those of security and protection, we seek to satisfy our need for love and above all for belonging, by achieving professional and occupational positioning as nurses, by belonging to the guild, to a civil, governmental or private organization; as we have already mentioned, we seek to satisfy our need for love and, above all, for belonging.

As mentioned in previous sections, nursing has the possibility of satisfying its needs and also of not satisfying them, this research aims to describe professional satisfaction in the field of nursing care.

If nursing cannot satisfy their needs for self-esteem and much less for self-fulfillment, the low quality of the care they could provide is foreseen and not only this is added, but feelings and sensations are produced that lead to the decadence of the self, Kozier (1998) comments that an individual with poor self-esteem may have unsatisfied all or part of their need for self-esteem; likewise an individual with an unsatisfied need for belonging may have problems in their professional performance (Maslow, Abraham, 1991).

Maslow (1943) then proposes, within his theory of personality, the concept of hierarchy of needs, in which needs are structurally organized with different degrees of power. Scale of needs by priority order in which we have physiological needs: activity, rest, food, elimination. Safety and security needs: feeling of security in their environment and relationships, covering physical and emotional aspects. The need for love and belonging: giving and receiving love, affection, affection and the need to feel part of a social group.

The need for self-esteem: the need to satisfy the demands of the functional pattern of health, self-image, self-concept and role-relationships. The need for self-fulfillment: encompasses the need to show the maximum innate potential, by satisfying this need one gets to satisfy all the other needs because one has found the object of one's whole life.

In living our own lives, human beings seek to satisfy our individual and peculiar needs; children, adults, seniors, under any marital status, sex, professional or not; Maslow's theory (1943) states that the lower needs are a priority, and therefore, more powerful than the higher needs in the hierarchy.

Only when the person succeeds in satisfying the lower needs, albeit relatively, do the higher needs gradually enter into his or her awareness, and with that the motivation to satisfy them; as the positive tendency becomes more important, a greater degree of psychological health is experienced, which is directly related to professional satisfaction, and a movement towards full humanization.
Maslow's theory can be applied to this research as follows
example that when you have professional satisfaction, you will find the
individual on the verge of achieving self-realization, this is secondary to the fact that
success, self-worth and prestige are indispensable elements of the
(Maslow, A Theory of Human Motivation and Motivation,
2012).

Nursing as a professional discipline, a work tool, an opportunity to transcend and perpetuate a knowledge and care, a way of life, and an indispensable resource for the health of populations, gives us the guideline to satisfy our entire scale of needs as long as it is lived with the right attitude and opportunities are sought, on the contrary it will facilitate personal, professional and labor dissatisfaction, as well as the frustration of various feelings that affect the health status of the professional and his quality of life.(Cifuentes, 2012).

Maslow's (1991) theories of motivation for work have been attractive as explanations of organizational behavior, since they have contributed to elucidate the reason why workers are productive and what drives their behavior, and because they have attempted to explain the direction that organizational behavior takes once it is activated (Contreras, 2013).

There is a classification proposed by Campbell, Dunnette, Lawler & Weick in 1973, described by Weinert (1985) and by many authors who study the subject of job satisfaction, which divides motivation theories into two groups: content or knowledge/cause theories and process theories. Process theories try to explain which factors guide human behavior, trying to identify which specific aspects and factors motivate people to work, in addition to the desires that move people to act and the needs they try to satisfy. For this reason they are also known as needs theories. These include: Maslow's hierarchy model; Alderfer's ERG theory. Process theories of work motivation emphasize how specific aspects and factors guide the individual to work in a certain way, and by what goals his work behavior is directed and determined. (Weinert, 1985).

These theories analyze which parameters can be modified to promote specific changes in work behavior, and many of them are complementary rather than competitive, basically consisting of the instrumentality or expectations theories and the equilibrium theories.

In his research, Herzberg (1959) assumed that job satisfaction has two dimensions: individual satisfaction and dissatisfaction. These dimensions are affected by two different groups of factors, i.e., the factors that generate satisfaction are different from those that produce dissatisfaction. Herzberg called these two groups or classes of job aspects: hygienic or extrinsic factors and motivational or intrinsic factors. The hygienic or extrinsic factors refer to the working conditions or that the environment contributes to the worker's task. These conditions are located in the external environment surrounding the individual, they are managed and decided by the company, therefore, hygienic factors are beyond the control of individuals.

The main extrinsic factors include: administrative organization (company policies and guidelines, work rules or internal regulations, work guidelines or procedures, type of direction or supervision that people receive from their superiors); salary; social benefits; complexity of the task; working hours; working conditions (physical and environmental working conditions, pleasant environment, safety at work, personal space); the climate of relations between the company and the people who work in it; social status, etc. (Herzberg, 2010).

Because of this more dissatisfaction-oriented influence, Herzberg calls them hygienic factors, since they are essentially prophylactic and preventive: they only prevent dissatisfaction but do not cause satisfaction. Their effect is similar to that of certain hygienic remedies: they prevent infection or combat headache, but do not improve health. Because they are more related to dissatisfaction, Herzberg also calls them dissatisfying factors.

The second group of factors are the so-called intrinsic or motivational factors, which are related to the content of the position and the nature of the tasks that the individual performs. These factors are under the control of the individual and are related to what he does and performs. They involve feelings of individual growth, professional recognition and self-fulfillment needs and depend on the tasks the individual performs in his job (Herzberg, 2010).

Intrinsic or motivational factors include work rhythm, autonomy, opinions, participation, work content, responsibility, achievement, progress, recognition, etc.

The effect of motivational factors on people's behavior is much deeper and more stable. Because they are linked to the satisfaction of individuals, Herzberg also calls them satisfying factors (Herzberg, 2010).

In this model, the existence of a double continuum is postulated between satisfaction and its opposite, non satisfaction and dissatisfaction and its opposite, non dissatisfaction. Thus, it is considered that work affects job satisfaction in two different ways: first, in relation to the presence or absence of certain motivating factors and second, by the so-called hygienic factors, as a series of working conditions that make possible an attractive work environment. (Herzberg, 2010).

That is to say, when hygiene factors are optimal or covered, they only prevent employee dissatisfaction, although they may not be motivated, since they do not manage to consciously raise satisfaction, and when they do raise it, they do not manage to sustain it for a long time. On the contrary, when hygiene factors are lacking, poor or precarious, they cause dissatisfaction.

In this sense, Herzberg (2010) states that extrinsic factors cannot determine job satisfaction; they can only prevent or avoid it when it exists. Motivational factors, on the other hand, when they are optimal, cause people's satisfaction; when they are precarious, they prevent satisfaction.

Based on this conclusion, Herzberg (2010) proposes two types of needs: Physiological needs, associated with hygiene factors and psychological needs associated with motivational factors.

Motivational factors are related to one's own behavior and its social acceptance, and are proposed as a scale differentiated from dissatisfaction, creating job satisfaction-motivation, by covering individual needs for growth and personal recognition. Therefore, once the hygienic factors have been controlled, the motivational factors would promote satisfaction and encourage productivity.

Research subsequent to Herzberg's (2010) found that the distinction between intrinsic and extrinsic factors is important and useful, and that there are significant individual differences in terms of the relative importance attached to one or the other factors.

Factors related to job satisfaction, the literature attaches great importance to theories of motivation and their relationship with the satisfaction that workers may or may not experience, raising points of convergence that show that these theories are not incompatible with each other.

In this sense, job satisfaction is conceived as a positive or pleasant emotional state (psychological states, expectations A and B), experienced by the worker in relation to the subjective perception of the subject's work experiences, influenced by the circumstances and characteristics of the work performed (extrinsic factors), and the individual characteristics of each worker (intrinsic factors).

Thus, a worker is considered to be satisfied with his job when, as a result of his work, he experiences feelings of well-being, pleasure or happiness; otherwise, the worker is not satisfied.

The results of a lack of satisfaction can affect the productivity of the organization and produce a deterioration in the quality of the work environment, decrease performance, increase the level of complaints, absenteeism or job change.

Therefore, the relationship between intrinsic and extrinsic aspects within a given context conditions the individual's affective response to different aspects of the job and is a determining factor in the quality of care.

EMPIRICAL FRAMEWORK

Taking into account the main concepts or variables of this research, the following studies were found:

At the international level:

Del Río Moro (2001) Spain, in their research Satisfaction of the Nursing Staff, makes a bibliographic review of the studies carried out on nursing and their job satisfaction in the last fourteen years. They conclude that what most satisfies nurses are interpersonal relationships and professional competence; what least satisfies them is salary, lack of promotion and training, distance from the workplace as an institution and poor working conditions (Del Río, 2001).

Izaguirre, C. (2004) in Honduras, studied the degree of job satisfaction among employees of the Metropolitan Health Region of Honduras, associating it with five facets of the job: the current job, salary, opportunities for promotion, supervision, work companionship and some biological and social characteristics of the workers. The main finding reflects that the job satisfaction of employees is associated more with the facets of the job itself and the salary, than with the biological and social characteristics of the workers (Izaguirre, Carlos; Reyes, Hermes, 2004).

Álvarez C. (2003) in Spain, whose study is called Motivación laboral (Work Motivation). in a hospital emergency department concluded that work motivation perceived by physicians, DUE/ATS and nursing assistants that work in the Emergency Department of the Cabueñes Hospital in Gijón, Spain, through five basic behavioral components: the level of activation and necessity, the value of each subject's incentive, the level of expectations, performance and satisfaction (Alvarez, 2002).

Briceño C. (2005) in Argentina. In his study "Job Satisfaction in Nursing Personnel in the Public Sector", he identified that ergonomic risks are related to job satisfaction and its incidence on the health of nursing workers, observing a high prevalence of pathologies, mainly in the female sex. Regarding the levels of job satisfaction, the analysis shows conformity in the type of work performed and the relationship with colleagues. Salary and promotion possibilities cause greater dissatisfaction. It also highlights the need to improve working conditions and reduce the high rate of occupational pathologies, incorporating preventive measures, control procedures, promotion of training programs and training of employees and quality of care for users (Briceño, 2005).

Ponce, G. (2006) in Mexico, a study in the Gynecology-Obstetrics Hospital No. 3 described the factors that intervene in the perception of the quality of nursing care and those that influence the nurse's job satisfaction. When comparing the variables, it was found that evening shift personnel and those with three jobs showed higher rates of dissatisfaction (Ponce, Reyes, and Ponce, 2006).

Gutiérrez, H. (2008) In Mexico, in the study "Satisfacción profesional del nursing care staff at different stages of development professional in public and private hospitals in Zamora, MIchoacan. hospital, where the objective was to identify the satisfiers of nursing through a quantitative study. Using the method questionnaire obtaining results for the data to be collected concluding that the rate of dissatisfaction was located in the presence of doctors

Laverde, A. (2008) in Colombia conducted a study on the performance and job satisfaction of the nursing staff in the Third Level of Care emergency service in the city of Medellin,

Colombia; they determine the condition of the physical environment, by intrinsic factors: amount of work, recognition received for performance, training and induction and among the extrinsic factors: acceptance of suggestions, physical structure, availability of resources and salary, as well as personal aspects: stress and overload. They point out that the relationship between colleagues is adequate and they feel satisfied with the comfort of the physical area, although in some aspects they are concerned about the lack of space and privacy to attend users, insecurity, functionality and equipment (Laverde, Forero, Pulido, & Macías, 2008).

The following factors were found to be the most important in the new surveys: 6.81% underestimation of nurses' knowledge, poor coordination among the health team, mistrust 9.09%, irresponsibility and negligence 25%, lack of support from colleagues in difficult situations with patients 22.72%, rotation through the services 11.36%, lack of material and human resources 15.90%, poor remuneration for the work 18.18% 8.

Fernández, B. (2008) in Chile conducted a research on the level of job satisfaction of nurses in public and private hospitals and identified some factors related to this satisfaction. It was found that the factors of dissatisfaction in both groups are: remuneration in 5.96% of public and 11.21% of private hospitals. Dissatisfaction with activities and promotions and/or promotions in 33.20% of public and 34.75% of private hospitals, and poor interaction with their superiors or bosses in 37.76% of public and 35.08% of private hospitals (Fernández, 2008).

Cifuentes, J. (2012) in Colombia whose study is entitled Job satisfaction in nursing in a fourth level of care health institution. An 80% participation rate was obtained. Nurses are those who present greater dissatisfaction in relation to men. Male nurses are more satisfied with their work, but present greater pressure and tension in relation to their work. Nurses who have been in their profession for more than 7 years are more dissatisfied with their work than those who have been in their profession for less time (Cifuentes, 2012).

Contreras, M. (2013) in Colombia in the study of Job Satisfaction of nursing professionals linked to an I.P.S of III level of care; the results of this study show that 58% of the population presents a medium level of job satisfaction. Followed by 31% of the population with a high level of job satisfaction and finally 11% of the population with a low level of job satisfaction, it could be said that job satisfaction in nursing is a multidimensional phenomenon that is conditioned by a variety of factors that affect job performance and the quality of services provided (Contreras, 2013).

Rufaza, M. (2017) in Spain, a study was conducted where it was allowed to evaluate the job satisfaction of Spanish nursing professionals, working in English hospitals and the influence of various labor partner variables, where nurses working in English hospitals have an average level of overall satisfaction in an average of 25.8%. Those associated with higher job satisfaction were relationships with colleagues and immediate bosses at 48.3%. The dimensions with lower job satisfaction were job satisfaction and professional competence at 12.5%. (Ruzafa, Torres, Velandrino, & Iborra, 2017).

At the national level:

Torres, C. (2008) in Peru conducted a study on the job satisfaction experienced by general nurses during the service of their profession at the E. Rebagliatti Hospital and Dos Mayo Hospital, and concluded that 65% of nurses experience job dissatisfaction and 35% satisfaction. The factors that determine job dissatisfaction are extrinsic: organization, salary and physical environment. Comparing job satisfaction among nurses in both institutions, it was found that in the E. Rebagliatti hospital 60% of the nurses experience job dissatisfaction, while in the Dos de Mayo hospital 90% of them experience job dissatisfaction in their professional practice (Torres, 2008).

JUSTIFICATION:

The nurse working in a surgical center has a preponderant role in the direct care of patients, both physically, psychologically and emotionally. Therefore, it is necessary to have an optimal environment with stable working conditions, since this could influence the quality of patient care.

In our reality, health personnel face different situations in their work, regarding treatment, working conditions, infrastructure, etc. When interacting with them it is common to hear: There is no recognition of the work we do, we do not have enough surgical material and instruments to be able to perform our work, the infrastructure is not adequate to develop our work, there are no training programs that allow us to improve, we do not have measures to protect our health, there is no recognition of my work, there is no training in the area, among other expressions.

The relevance and justification of the study to be investigated is the job satisfaction of the health personnel of the Regional Teaching Hospital of Trujillo, in order to find criteria to facilitate decision making that will show as consequences an improvement in the daily practice of the new professionals, an observable improvement in the quality of life, health status and human relations of the health personnel and evidently in the quality of professional care.

It is the duty of all health professionals to fully identify with the profession, otherwise negative feelings arise that have repercussions on the absence of harmony in the biopsycho-spiritual environment, so this research yields results that help in the motivational and participatory processes in the work and training centers, since it is an institution that provides services and at the same time trains professionals in various disciplines in the field of health.

At present, in the surgical center of the Regional Teaching Hospital of Trujillo there is a climate of demotivation, tension and daily confrontations due to the lack of supplies, materials and equipment for direct patient care such as bed linen, anesthesia machines, problems in the sterilization process, lack of personnel, among others; all these inconveniences are daily causes of tension situations that make the health personnel confront with relatives, surgeons and other actors involved in the different operative times.

For this reason, the following question was posed:

Is there a relationship between working conditions and the level of job satisfaction of health personnel in the surgical center of the Hospital Regional Docente de Trujillo January - February 2016?

GENERAL OBJECTIVE

- To determine the relationship between working conditions and job satisfaction of health personnel of Centro Quirúrgico del Hospital Regional Docente de Trujillo period January - February 2016.

SPECIFIC OBJECTIVES:

- To determine the working conditions of the health personnel of the Surgical Center of the Regional Teaching Hospital of Trujillo, January-February 2016.

- To determine the job satisfaction of the health personnel of Centro Quirúrgico del Hospital Regional Docente de Trujillo period January-February 2016.

Chapter 2
II.MATERIAL AND METHOD

II.1. TYPE OF RESEARCH

The present work is a quantitative research, of a descriptive correlational type, of transversal cut, since variables were studied simultaneously at a certain moment making a cut in time and descriptive since it allowed to create a systematic guide to determine solutions and to know in correlational form the variables (Jimenez, R, 1998).

This study was conducted at the Surgical Center Service of the Hospital Regional Docente de Trujillo during the months of January and February 2016.

II.2. STUDY POPULATION AND SAMPLE

II.2.1. Sample Universe

The sample universe consisted of all health personnel working in the surgical center service of the Regional Teaching Hospital of Trujillo, applied to doctors, nurses, nursing technicians, which corresponds to a total of 51 health workers, between the three shifts, during the months of January and February 2016.

II.3. Analysis Unit

The unit of analysis was constituted by the health personnel working in the Surgical

Center of the Regional Teaching Hospital of Trujillo: it was applied to physicians, nurses and nursing technicians who met the inclusion and exclusion criteria.

II.3.1. Inclusion criteria

a) Nurses, physicians and nursing technicians working in the Surgical Center with a minimum service time of 6 months.

b) Nurses, physicians, and nursing technicians who agreed to voluntarily participate in the research study.

II.3.2. Exclusion Criteria

Nurses, physicians, and nursing technicians who were not on duty due to leave of absence, furlough, and/or vacation during the research study.

II.4. Study Scenario

The setting for the present study was the surgical center service of the Hospital Regional Docente de Trujillo, during the months of January and February 2016.

II.5. Instruments

Two instruments were used for data collection:

II.5.1. EVALUATION OF WORKING CONDITIONS

The measurement instrument used was the evaluation of working conditions developed by the authors: Juan Carlos García Ubaque, Alejandra Husley Beltrán Lizarazo, Magda Liliana Daza López (2011) and modified by the author (Annex 01).

It is a self-administered scale, composed of 47 items that assesses the variable working conditions, presenting for each item two answers, which are: yes or no, depending on the type of question, the answer would correspond to be acceptable and white or risky and lead color, as shown below:

Working condition Acceptable	0
Work Condition at Risk	1

Once the information was obtained and qualified, the evaluation of working conditions of health personnel was classified as follows:

- **Acceptable working conditions**: 0 to 24 points.

- **Working conditions at risk**: 25 - 48 points.

This instrument was used taking into account only the score obtained at the end, but the sub-classification was not taken into account.

II.5.2. JOB SATISFACTION QUESTIONNAIRE

The Font Roja questionnaire instrument on job satisfaction developed by Mary Luz Contreras Contreras, Bogotá 2013, modified by the author, was used; the instrument consists of 24 items (Annex 02).

This author established contact with the person who validated the instrument in Colombia, Dr. Fred Manrique, demonstrating its validity and reliability with a Crombach's alpha = 0.7683.

It was answered with an ordinal Likert-type scale ranging from 0 to 5, the range of scores for the entire questionnaire goes from 24 (minimum degree of job satisfaction) to 120 (maximum degree of job satisfaction) as follows:

1	2	3	4	5
Very agreement	Agreed	Neither agree nien disagreement	At disagreement	Strongly disagree

The use of the Font Roja questionnaire in this research will be based on the analysis of job satisfaction, taking into account the scores achieved by the responses of each participant, i.e. the total sum of the score obtained.

To establish the cut-off points for the Font Roja instrument, the Dalenius rule was used. The measurement scale used to define the cut-off points suggests three stratification categories for the interpretation of this instrument:

a) Low level of job satisfaction between 89 - 120 points on the scale.

b) Average level of job satisfaction scores between 57 - 88 points on the scale.

c) High level of job satisfaction with scores between 24 - 56 points on the scale.

II.6. Quality control of instruments

II.6.1. Pilot Test

The instruments of the present investigation were applied in the Hospital Belén de Trujillo with the health personnel of the Surgical Center, with a total of 17 participants who had similar characteristics to the study population, who will not be considered in the sample universe. This was done in order to know their understanding, practicality and time of application of these instruments, as well as to provide the necessary basis for the reliability of the same.

II.6.2. Validity and Reliability

Validity: the instruments considered for this research are instruments already validated by their authors, such that the instrument Test: Working Conditions is an instrument developed by Nelson Hernández (2011), and adapted by García U. (2011).

The other instrument is Cuestionario Sobre Satisfacción Laboral, the Font Roja questionnaire instrument on job satisfaction developed by Mary Luz Contreras Contreras Contreras Bogotá 2013 was used, the instrument consists of 24 items.

Reliability: To evaluate the reliability of the instruments, the instruments were applied to the pilot sample and subsequently Cronbach's alpha coefficient was evaluated for each of them.

The values obtained are:

Reliability Analysis for Test: TEST CONDITIONS

Cronbach's alpha	0.81
N° of items	48
No. of persons	17

WORK (Garcia J. 2011).

Cronbach's alpha	0.734
N° of items	24
No. of persons	17

Reliability Analysis for Test: Level of Satisfaction

Labor o FONT ROJA QUESTIONNAIRE (Contreras M. 2013)

An instrument is considered reliable when its Cronbach's alpha coefficient is at least 0.70; from the above it can be said that the instruments are reliable.

II.7. Procedure

a) In order to carry out this research study, authorization was requested from the management of the Regional Teaching Hospitals of Trujillo and Belén, both of which belong to MINSA and have similar conditions. Subsequently, coordination was made with the Head Nurse of the Department, in order to allow the application of the instruments of the present study.

b) Health personnel meeting the inclusion and exclusion criteria were selected.

c) The instruments were then applied, using the personal interview technique in 30 minutes; the objectives, purpose of the study, the form of response and/or qualification of each instrument were previously informed. The answers were filled out by the participants themselves for their convenience.

d) The instruments were applied every day of the week until the sample was complete.

e) The ethical principles of confidentiality, informed consent, human dignity, respect and free participation were taken into account in this research.

II.8. Data Processing and Analysis

The data processing was carried out using the Working Conditions Evaluation and Font Roja Questionnaire instruments, which were then entered into a spreadsheet (Excel) and processed using the IBM statistical program SPSS STATISTIC 23.

The results are presented in single- and double-entry tables with their respective graphs, according to the proposed objectives.

The statistical analysis used the Chi-Square Test of Independence of Criteria (x^2), to see if there is a relationship between variables, considering a level of statistical significance if the probability is less than 5 percent ($p < 0.05$).

II.9. Research Ethics

The following ethical principles were taken into account in this study:

a) Confidentiality

It will be explained to the health personnel about the research study, which will be kept secret. (Avila, J, 2013).

b) Informed Consent

That the participants voluntarily agree to participate in the research (University of Chile Interdisciplinary Center for Bioethics Studies, 1994).

c) Respect for Human Dignity

The objectives of the research were explained to the health personnel and their decision to voluntarily participate in this research was respected (León, Francisco, 2017).

II.10. Definition of Variables

a.- Dependent Variable: **WORKING CONDITIONS**

- **Nominal definition**: working conditions and environment are inherent to the work process and refer to "the set of factors that act on the individual in a work situation, determining his activity and causing a series of consequences both for the individual himself (human costs) and for the company (economic costs)" (Cifuentes R. 2012).

- **Operational definition:** I used the scores obtained from the sum of the items applied. Determining: **Acceptable Working Conditions: 0 to 24 points**

Working Conditions at Risk: 25 - 48 points.

b. Independent variable: JOB SATISFACTION.

- **Nominal Definition**: It is the attitude with which the worker faces his own work. This attitude based on the beliefs and values that the worker develops about his own work is determined, jointly, by the current characteristics of the job with the perceptions that the worker has of what it should be (Jaramillo Y 2010).

- **Operational definition**:

The stratification categories for the interpretation of this instrument are:

Low level of job satisfaction between 89 - 120 points.

Average level of job satisfaction between 57 - 88 points.

High job satisfaction level of 24 - 56 points.

RESULTS

TABLE N° 01

WORKING CONDITIONS OF HEALTH PERSONNEL AT THE SURGICAL CENTER OF THE SURGICAL CENTER OF THE REGIONAL TEACHING HOSPITAL OF TRUJILLO, JANUARY - FEBRUARY 2016.

Working Conditions	N°	%
Acceptable	37	72.5
At Risk	14	27.5
Total	51	100.0

Source: Information obtained from instruments applied to HRDT surgical center health personnel.

CHART N° 1

WORKING CONDITIONS OF HEALTH CARE PERSONNEL AT THE SURGICAL CENTER OF THE REGIONAL TEACHING HOSPITAL

OF TRUJILLO, JANUARY - FEBRUARY 2016.

Source: Information obtained from the instruments applied to the health personnel of the HRDT surgical center.

TABLE N° 02

LEVEL OF JOB SATISFACTION OF HEALTH PERSONNEL OF THE SURGICAL CENTER OF THE REGIONAL TEACHING HOSPITAL OF TRUJILLO, JANUARY - FEBRUARY 2016.

Satisfaction Level Laboral	N°	%
High	2	3.9
Medium	40	78.4
Under	9	17.6
Total	51	100.0

Source: Information obtained from instruments applied to HRDT surgical center health personnel.

CHART N° 02

**LEVEL OF JOB SATISFACTION OF
HEALTH PERSONNEL OF THE SURGICAL CENTER OF THE
REGIONAL TEACHING
HOSPITAL**

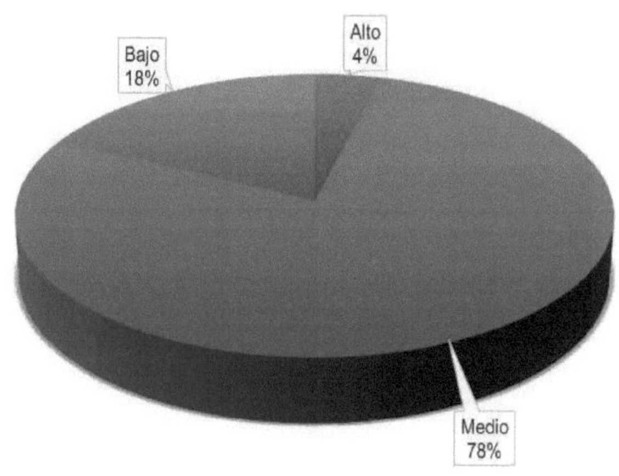

**OF TRUJILLO, JANUARY - FEBRUARY
2016.**

Source: Information obtained from instruments applied to HRDT surgical center health personnel.

TABLE N° 03

RELATIONSHIP BETWEEN WORKING CONDITIONS AND THE LEVEL OF JOB SATISFACTION AMONG

JOB SATISFACTION OF HEALTH PERSONNEL IN THE SURGICAL CENTER SURGICAL CENTER OF THE REGIONAL TEACHING HOSPITAL OF TRUJILLO, JANUARY - FEBRUARY 2016.

	LEVEL	I WAS SATISFIED LABORAL	XION	
CONDITIONS OF WORK	Under	Medium	High	Total
	N° %	N° %	N° %	
Acceptable	38.1	3286 .5	2 5.4	37
At Risk	6 42.9	1 857.	0 0.0	14
Total	9 17.6	4078 .4	2 3.9	51

X2P

8.8220 .0121

Source: Information obtained from instruments applied to HRDT surgical center health personnel.

CHART N° 03
R ELATION BETWEEN WORKING CONDITIONS AND THE LEVEL OF JOB SATISFACTION OF HEALTH PERSONNEL IN THE SURGICAL CENTER AREA OF THE REGIONAL TEACHING HOSPITAL OF TRUJILLO, JANUARY - FEBRUARY, 2009. 2016.

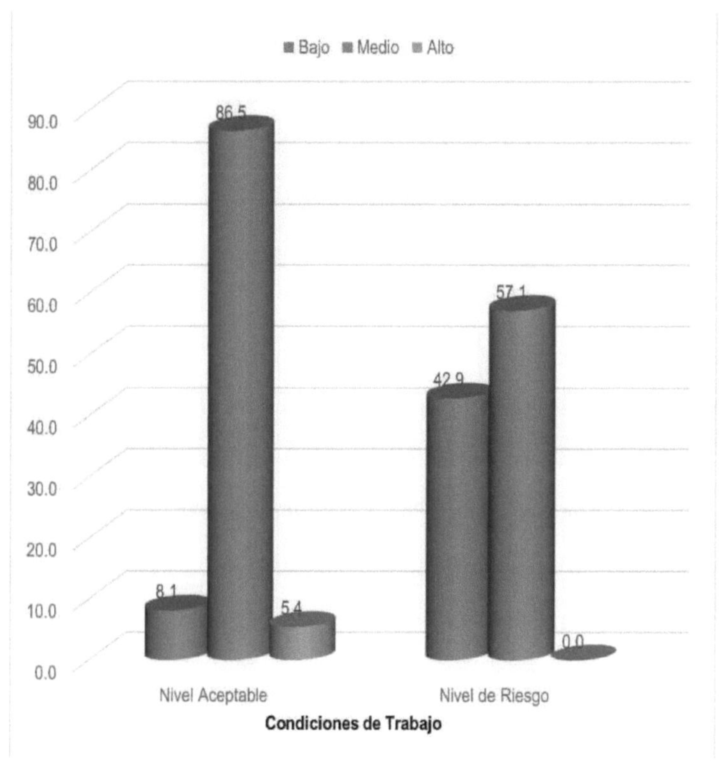

Source: Information obtained from instruments applied to HRDT surgical center health personnel.

Chapter 3
III. ANALYSIS AND DISCUSSION

Table N°01 and Graph N°01:

It is observed that 73% of the health personnel have an acceptable level of working conditions, compared to 27% who have a risk level. As can be noted from the presentation of the results of this research, a matter of concern is the null percentage obtained for the item referring to optimal working conditions in the workers of the Surgical Center service of the Regional Teaching Hospital, since it is only observed that 73% of the referred health personnel present an acceptable level of working conditions, compared to 27% who have a risk level.

This should be analyzed in the light of the theories presented in the theoretical framework of the thesis report, since, according to these theories, there is a close relationship between the working conditions of the workers and their satisfaction with the work itself and with their work center; finally, this interrelationship has a direct influence on the efficiency at the time of performing their duties and, consequently, on the care provided to the users of the health sector.

The concern about the absence of the optimum in the working conditions of workers was mentioned because, despite the arbitrariness that may be present in the so-called individual or extrinsic conditions, it is very relevant to observe the intrinsic conditions related to the workplace, infrastructure, tools, training, work incentives, among others, which, at least, could create a pleasant working environment and greatly favor worker satisfaction.

Thus, when it is observed that the working conditions in the work center are not optimal, but only acceptable, the worker's possibility of having a positive or pleasant emotional state resulting from the subjective perception of positive work experiences is directly affected; this keeps the worker at an average level of satisfaction and, consequently, the hygiene factors of the work scenario remain stabilized, but the motivational factors are disadvantaged.

It should be taken into account that motivational factors are the main ingredient to achieve worker's job satisfaction and, thus, the efficient attention of health sector users, which is the main purpose of this sector.

On the other hand, it is worth mentioning that this problem is present in most public establishments because the personnel are generally not identified with the service techniques as much as with the techniques of their work, the administrative part does not promote workshops, training, humanitarian situations, but merely technical-professional situations, which ends up causing this average situation of labor comfort, technical compliance but not organizational.

Without wishing to draw conclusions about the interrelation between the elements studied, a first assertion can be made that the percentages obtained regarding the acceptable level of working conditions (73%), which shows a regular situation of conditions in the hospital, as well as the risk level of working conditions (27%), which specifies an important figure of total deficiency of conditions; Together, they show that in the hospital there is a situation of medium compliance with the physiological needs of the workers, but that there is no compliance with the psychological needs that contribute so much to the positive evolution of health care.

It should be clarified that the level of risk has been assessed in a fundamental way because it is the result of the poor conditions that depend directly on the hospital administration, among which are the quality of family life, travel time to get to the work center, with the exception of the lack of recognition of the work by the representatives of the health entity referred to by the workers.

Table N°02 and Graph N°02

It is observed that 18% of the health personnel have a low level of job satisfaction, 78% have a medium level, and only 4% have a high level of job satisfaction.

In accordance with what was outlined in the previous section, the level of satisfaction of the workers of the Surgical Center of the Teaching Hospital of Trujillo is also presented; 18% of the health personnel have a low level of job satisfaction, which implies that there are workers who are not satisfied with the intrinsic elements of their work, i.e., the hospital infrastructure, the instruments provided to them to perform their work, schedules, organization, among others; This is compounded by the personal problems they have and the extrinsic ones, such as the distance between their homes and their work center, the need for mobility, social factors, among others.

As in the results obtained in the previous section, there is a significant percentage of workers who are moderately satisfied with their work and their work center; this percentage amounts to 78% of workers and, contrary to what one might think, this is a discouraging figure, because, as has been supported in the theoretical framework, these average levels of satisfaction mean that workers are only satisfied with the status quo at work but do not produce or contribute significantly to their work, As has been argued in the theoretical framework, these average levels of satisfaction mean that workers are only satisfied with the *status quo* at work but do not produce or contribute significantly to the work of the company, in this case, the public entity.

It should be remembered that a hospital is a public center that depends on the Regional Health Directorate and this, in turn, on the Regional Government, a governmental entity whose task is to execute one of the primary functions of the Executive Power, that is, to promote the population's right to health through the administration of health policies and activities aimed at providing this service, which are very important because they make effective a social right considered fundamental for the human being.

This means that the service provided by the health sector must be of high quality, efficient with respect to the workers and effective with respect to the policies and activities deployed; consequently, if there is no motivational work environment for the workers, they will not produce enough to perform their tasks efficiently, and this will ultimately affect the health service provided by the hospital itself.

Therefore, this important percentage (78%) should go from a medium level of satisfaction to a high level of satisfaction of workers with their work and their work center, which is currently only 4%, a percentage that indicates that there is a small number of workers satisfied with what they do and that customer service is only efficient and effective to a lesser degree.

Thus, the medium level of satisfaction, according to the theories indicated in the theoretical framework, produces conformism, fatigue, monotony in the work center and in the workers; the high level of satisfaction, on the other hand, produces a positive or pleasant emotional state, which favors the performance of the work itself and has a direct effect on the correct execution of the health service; thus, this aspect should be improved in the Teaching Hospital of Trujillo.

Table N° 03 and Graph N° 03

It is observed that there is a significant relationship between both variables, when applying the Chi-square test a high degree of significance of 0.0121 is observed; concluding that 87% of the health personnel present acceptable working conditions and at the same time a medium level of job satisfaction, and 42.9% of the health personnel present risky working conditions and at the same time a low level of job satisfaction.

These crossed results between the working conditions and the satisfaction of the workers of the Surgical Center of the Teaching Hospital of Trujillo constitute the core of the work, since they have verified the influence that the working conditions have on the satisfaction of the workers and, finally, these two aspects on the efficiency and effectiveness in the execution of the health service in this hospital.

In the first place, 87% of the health personnel have an acceptable level of working conditions and at the same time an average level of job satisfaction; this, as previously stated, in accordance with Maslow's personality theory, the working conditions available to the workers of the Surgical Center of the Teaching Hospital of Trujillo do not fully cover their needs such as physiological needs related to activity, rest, food, elimination; the need for security and protection: feeling of security in their environment and their relationships; the need for love and belonging: giving and receiving love, affection, affection and the need to feel part of a social group; the need for self-esteem: need to satisfy the demands of the functional pattern of health self-image self-concept and role relationships; the need for self-realization: to show the maximum innate potential, by satisfying this need one gets to satisfy all the others because one has found the object of one's whole life; among others.

We can also mention that in this hospital the health personnel have to work with a population of low economic resources, and this institution belongs to the Ministry of Health, an entity that provides supplies and work materials in a scarce and untimely manner, which is reflected in job dissatisfaction, so often they have to work in conditions that put the health of workers and patients at risk. As a result, the staff feels that they do not have adequate conditions to work, generating job dissatisfaction.

The medium level of satisfaction, in the specific case, is related to the fact that the aforementioned hospital workers effectively have physiological factors that scarcely cover their needs of the same type, such as infrastructure, equipment, technical training, among others; and lack other elements that would favor their psychological needs, such as incentives, recognition, psychological workshops, good treatment, organizational work, medical controls or check-ups, among others.

Consequently, this proportion of merely objective factors to the workers disfavors their technical performance and keeps them in a state of conformism that does not contribute anything to the motivational and participative processes in the work centers and affects the user's attention as a service provider institution.

So much so that 42.9% of health personnel have a risk level of working conditions and at the same time a low level of job satisfaction; an important percentage that puts the health service itself at risk and should be alleviated as soon as possible. Adequate measures should be taken to improve working conditions by the authorities and other social actors of the health services. Health personnel have to face this situation every day and many times they feel powerless because they cannot provide the best care to the user due to the lack of supplies and materials they need.

This result is believed to be because currently in all hospitals of the Ministry of Health is going through a crisis so marked that is reflected in the quality of direct patient care, facing so many patients and inadequate conditions, this is coupled with overcrowding in the services, the urgent need for emergency surgery, which causes stress and dissatisfaction at the same time.

CONCLUSIONS

- It is concluded that 7 percent of the health personnel have acceptable working conditions and 27.5 percent have risky working conditions; out of a population of 51 people.

- It is concluded that 78.4 percent of health personnel have a medium level of job satisfaction; and 3.9 percent of health personnel have a high level of job satisfaction, out of a population of 51 people.

- It is observed that there is a significant relationship between both variables, when applying the Chi-square statistical test, obtaining a result of $p < 0.0121$.

RECOMMENDATIONS

1. That this study serves to reflect on the job satisfaction of health personnel in institutions providing services of the Ministry of Health, since in many hospitals the personnel are not completely satisfied in their work due to work overload, low salaries, few training incentives and others.

2. The Ministry of Health should improve the working conditions of health personnel, in terms of personal protection, infrastructure and work overload.

3. That the competent authorities manage improvements in infrastructure, professional benefits for the personnel working in the institution under study.

4. Continue to conduct research and propose continuous improvements in order to provide adequate attention to the users of the institution under study.

5. Continuous training for health personnel according to the areas where they work, financed by the institution itself, especially on issues of work-related stress.
6. The nursing management should continue with the current policies, giving orientation to the service, creating motivation strategies: formation of high performance teams, which allows for continuous improvement and personal and professional growth.

7. The management should implement a training program on the development of emotional intelligence, as well as resume the induction courses for personnel and the talks assigned to professionals, review and modify the current system for selecting employees for training and courses, so that the choice of training is objective and equitable.

8. Managers are urged to allow proactive employee participation and make certain decisions

regarding teamwork in order to implement a culture of autonomy, strengthen communication, human relations and conflict management in an assertive manner and increase satisfaction within the company.

9. For subsequent studies of the same nature, it is recommended that the type of population, i.e., physicians, nurses and nursing technicians, be separated in order to obtain more specific data regarding the study conducted.

BIBLIOGRAPHIC REFERENCES

Avila, J. (October 20, 2013). *NATIONAL INSTITUTE OF SCIENCES MÉDICAS Y NUTRICIÓN SALVADOR ZUBIRÁN, MÉXICO.* Retrieved from http://www.innsz.mx/opencms/contenido/investigacion/comiteEtica/confidencialidadInformacion.html: http://www.innsz.mx/opencms/contenido/investigacion/comiteEtica/confidencialityInformation.html

Alvarez, C. (2002). *Work motivation in a hospital emergency department.* Spain.

Briceño, C. (2005). Job satisfaction in public sector nurses. *Electronic Journal of Intensive Care Medicine*, 50-62.

Calderon, A. (1999). *Absenteeism and degree of satisfaction of professionals in public administration.* Spain: Inmaculada.

Cardoso, M. (2013). *Absenteeism and its relationship with job satisfaction in nursing.* Madrid: Trotta.

Cifuentes, J. (2012). *Job satisfaction in nursing in a fourth level health care institution.* Bogotá: Universidad Nacional de Colombia.

Economic Commission for Latin America and the Caribbean (2009). Bulletin: ECLAC/ILO Report.

ECLAC/ILO Report, 20.

Contreras, M. (2013). *Master's Thesis in Nursing with emphasis in Nursing Management. Health Services and Nursing. Job satisfaction of nursing professionals linked to an I.P.S. of III level of care.* Bogota: National University of Colombia.

Del Río, O. (2001). *Personal nursing satisfaction: Are our expectations being met?* Madrid: 4th National Cardiology Congress.

Fernández, B. (2008). *Level of satisfaction of nurses in public and private hospitals in the Province of Concepción.* Concepción: University of Concepción.

García, J., Beltrán, A., & Daza, M. (2011). *Self-assessment of nursing working conditions in high complexity.* Bogotá: Universidad Nacional de Colombia.

Georgina, H. (2011). *Job Satisfaction Research Paper.* Argentina.

Gutiérrez, H. (2008). *Professional satisfaction of nursing personnel in the different stages of professional development in public and private hospitals in Zamora Michoacán. Graduate work. Nursing Department.* Zamora: School of Nursing, University of Zamora.

Hernandez, V. (2009). Motivation, job satisfaction, leadership and its relationship with service quality. *Cuban Journal of Military Medicine, vol. 38 no. 1*, 1-8.

Herzberg, F. (2010). *Teoría de los dos factores.* Lima: PUCP.

Izaguirre, Carlos; Reyes, Hermes (2004). *Job Satisfaction in the employees of the Metropolitan Sanitary Region, Tegucigalpa, M.D,C., Honduras C.A., I semester, Year 2004.* Honduras.

Jaramillo, Y., & Mendoza, M. (2010). *Degree dissertation for the Bachelor's Degree in Nursing. Job satisfaction of the nurse.*
Internal Medicine Service. Hospital (IVSS) "Dr. Hector Nouel Joubert". Bogotá: National University of Colombia.

Jimenez, R. (1998). *Research Methodology. Basic elements for clinical research.* Havana: Editorial Ciencias Médicas.

Laverde, A., Forero, L., Pulido, C., & Macías, G. (2008). Nursing staff management in the emergency department at a tertiary level clinic. *Journal of Educational Research in Nursing*, 112125.

León, Francisco (2017). Human Dignity, Freedom and Bioethics. *Grupo de Investigación en Bioética de Galicia de la UNIversidad de la Sabana.*

Maslow, A. (2012). *A theory and human motivations.* Lima: PUCP.

Maslow, Abraham (1991). *Motivación y personalidad.* Spain: Ediciones Díaz de Santos.

Robbins, S. (2004). *Organizational Behavior. 10th ed.* Mexico: Persons Prentice Hall.

Ruzafa, M., Torres, M., Velandrino, A., & Iborra, L. (October 12, 2017). *Job satisfaction of Spanish nursing professionals working in English hospitals*. Retrieved from Job satisfaction of Spanish nursing professionals working in English hospitals: http://scielo.org.br

Torres, C. (2008). *Job satisfaction experienced by general nurses during the service of their profession at the Edgardo Rebagliatti Hospital and Dos de Mayo Hospital during their professional practice.* Lima: PUCP.

University of Chile Interdisciplinary Center for Bioethics Studies (1994). *International Ethical Guidelines for Research and Experimentation biomedical research in humans.* Retrieved from h: ttp://www.uchile.cl/portal/investigacion/centro-interdisciplinario-de- studies-in-bioethics/documents/76203/the-guidelines-1-9-informed-consent

National University of Colombia (2008). *Gestión integral de la salud ocupación en a HUN - Conceptos generales (consultancy report).* Bogotá: Universidad Nacional de Colombia.

Viamontes, D. G. (2010). A Theoretical Approach . *Contribution to the Social Sciences.*

Weinert, A. (1985). *Handbook of Organizational Psychology. La conducta humana en las organizaciones.* Spain: Herder.

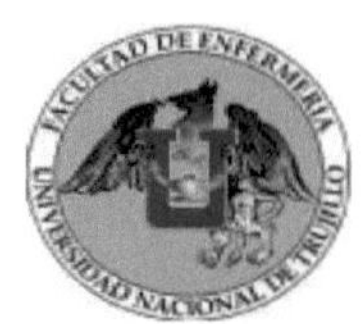

AMEXOS

ANNEX N° 01

NATIONAL UNIVERSITY OF TRUJILLO

FACULTY OF NURSING

EVALUATION OF WORKING CONDITIONS

Author: García J. (2011)

Adapted by López, A (2016)

Dear Mr. (a) Mr. (a) Miss Read carefully this questionnaire, which consists of several short questions, which gives you the opportunity to express your feelings in the area where you work. There are two possible answers, for which you have to mark with a cross the answer you think is correct in the yes or no box.

Indicate with a cross the answer you think is best, choose one, and only ONE answer for each question. This is not a test: there are no right or wrong answers. Please make an ASPA on the answer you think is best for each question.

1 Which of these statements best describes your usual behavior?	Yes	Impatient, irritable, dominant, very competitive.
	No	
	Yes	Calm, confident, with listening skills.
	No	
2 Is your physical health good?		Yes
		No
3 Is your mental health good?		Yes
		No
4 Does your job satisfy, at an acceptable level, your physiological, safety, social, esteem and fulfillment needs?		Yes
		No
5 Do you feel that the tasks you perform at work require more knowledge, experience and skills than you currently possess?		Yes
		No

6 Do you consider that you are good at learning new things?		Yes
		No
7 Do you have a good self-concept and self-image?		Yes
		No
8 Are you able to communicate with other colleagues and learn from their experiences?		Yes
		No
9 Do you feel that there is often conflict with your beliefs and values at work?		Yes
		No
10 Does your work in the service meet the expectations you set in your training?		Yes
		No
11 Do you prefer not to make decisions at work and have a superior tell you what to do, in what order to proceed and how to act?		Yes
		No
12 Do you believe that the ventilation in your workplace is adequate?		Yes
		No
13 Is the lighting in your workplace adequate?		Yes
		No
14 Is your workstation oriented in such a way as to avoid reflections or shadows?		Yes
		No
15 During the work shift do you experience sudden changes in temperature?		Yes
		No
16 Has the use of sodium hypochlorite, chlorhexidine, alcohol or other chemicals produced any reaction in your body?		Yes
		No
17 Are containers with chemicals properly labeled?		Yes
		No
18 Do you understand the consequences of exposure to chemicals used in the service?		Yes
		No
19 Do you understand the consequences of being exposed to viruses, bacteria and fungi in your workplace?		Yes
		No

20 Do you know and apply the guidelines and protocols for handling biological substances in your workplace?		Yes
		No
21 Are risk protection measures used during the shift?		Yes
		No
22 Are you vaccinated against HBV and tetanus?		Yes
		No
23 Do you consider your work to be monotonous and repetitive?		Yes
		No
24 Do you feel satisfied with the tasks you perform at your workplace?		Yes
		No
25 During the work shift do you spend most of your time in uncomfortable positions?		Yes
		No
26 Do you have to lift any type of load beyond your capabilities?		Yes
		No
27 Are there sufficient personal protection measures during the work shift?		Yes
		No
28 Do you understand and implement the standard measures in the execution of the procedures performed in the surgical center?		Yes
		No
29 Are there waste containers close to the sites where you operate?		Yes
		No
30 Is the workspace clean, tidy, free of obstacles and with the necessary equipment?		Yes
		No
31 Do you have sufficient surveillance and accompaniment at your place of work?		Yes
		No
32 Do you often have to work longer hours or perform additional activities than agreed upon?		Yes
		No
33 Do you consider that your work is recognized by the representatives of the health entity?		Yes
		No

34 How would you rate your current employment relationship with the health care provider?		Stable
		Unstable
35 How would you rate your current income from work?		Fair and equitable
		Unfair or inequitable
36. Relationships with peers and superiors can be considered to be		Cordial and constructive
		Tense or difficult
37 Do you think your family's quality of life is good?		Yes
		No
38 Do you live in a rented apartment?		Yes
		No
39 Does the place where you live have all public services (electricity, water, basic sanitation and garbage collection)?		Yes
		No
40 Is the area where you live safe?		Yes
		No
41 Do you spend more than 1 hour commuting to and from work?		Yes
		No
42 How many children do you have?		2 or less
		3 or more
43 Is any member of your household unemployed, underemployed or informally employed?		Yes
		No
44 Does any member of your family have chronic illnesses or permanent disability conditions?		Yes
		No
45 Do you consider that your family is well protected in case of any contingency?		Yes
		No
46 Is your family affiliated to the different social protection systems?		Yes
		No
47 Do you have sufficient social, state and community support in case of need?		Yes
		No

Thank you for completing the questionnaire.

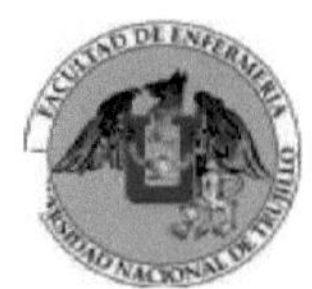

ANNEX N° 02

NATIONAL UNIVERSITY OF TRUJILLO

FACULTY OF NURSING

FONT ROJA QUESTIONNAIRE

Author: Aranaz J and Mira J. (1988)

Validated by Moya S. (2011)

Adapted by López, A (2016)

Dear colleague:

The work I have to do is an applied research on job satisfaction in health personnel, that is why I need your collaboration by answering the following questionnaire attached, which will not take you much time.

Please make a small effort to answer all questions honestly and thank you in advance.

The personal opinions collected in the questionnaire are strictly confidential. The overall results will be available to anyone who wishes to consult them.

Instructions

The Font Roja questionnaire contains a series of questions about your job and how you feel about it.

In no case are there correct, adequate or inadequate answers. What is important is your opinion on each of the questions/phrases and that opinion is always correct.

The response to the questionnaire is completely anonymous.

Taking into account the answer that most closely matches your opinion about what you are being asked, mark with a cross in the corresponding box based on the following scale:

1	2	3	4	5
Very much in agreement	Agreed	Neither agree nor disagree	Disagree	Strongly disagree

N°	QUESTIONS	Very much in agreement	Agreed	Neither agree No disagreement	At disagreement	Strongly disagree
		1	2	3	4	5
1	My current job at the hospital is the same every day, it never varies.					
2	I believe I have little responsibility for my work at the hospital.					
3	At the end of a normal workday, I am usually very tired.					
4	Quite often I have caught myself outside the hospital thinking about issues related to my work.					
5	Very few times I have been forced to use "full throttle" all my energy and capacity to do my job.					
6	Very rarely does my work at the hospital disturb my mood, or my health, or my sleep.					
7	I am very satisfied in my job.					
8	I have very little independence to organize the work I do, depending on my specific position.					
9	I have few opportunities to learn new things.					
10	I have very little interest in the things I do in my job.					
11	I have the feeling that what I am doing is not worth it.					
12	Generally, the recognition I get for my work is very comforting.					
13	The relationship with my bosses is very cordial.					
14	Relations with my colleagues are very cordial.					
15	The salary I receive is very adequate.					
16	I am convinced that the position I occupy is the one that really corresponds to my capacity and preparation.					
17	I have many opportunities for career advancement.					
18	I often have the feeling that there is not enough time to do my job.					
19	I am confident that I know what is expected of me by my managers.					
20	I think my workload is too much, I can't keep up with all the things that need to be done.					

21	The personal problems of my co-workers usually affect me.					
22	I often have the feeling that I am not qualified to do my job.					
23	I often feel that I do not have enough resources to do my job as well as I would like.					
24	Competitiveness, or keeping up with others, in my job often causes me stress or tension.					

THANK YOU VERY MUCH FOR YOUR COOPERATION AND TIME

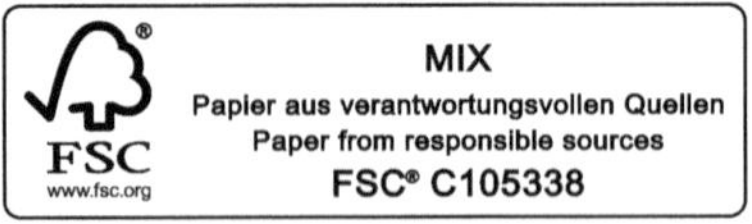

Printed by Books on Demand GmbH, Norderstedt / Germany